Comprehensive Safety Guide:
3 Books in 1

I0419787

Behavior Based Safety
+
Employee Safety and
Building Security
+
Reference Handbook of
Safety Risks

Louis Bevoc

Published by
NutriNiche System LLC

Louis Bevoc books...simple explanations of complex subjects

Behavior Based Safety
in Manufacturing
A Basic Introduction

Louis Bevoc

Published by
NutriNiche System LLC

Louis Bevoc books...simple explanations of complex subjects

Introduction

Safety has long been a concern of management and workers in manufacturing facilities because injuries cost a lot of money. More importantly, some injuries cause production workers pain and suffering that cannot be alleviated with monetary compensation because no amount of money is worth the loss of health that cannot be restored.

The above paragraph is true, but it leads to a question. If safety is a concern, then why do some manufacturing employees expose themselves to risks that could endanger their health and well-being? Sometimes it is because supervisors coerce them to behave unsafely. However, this type of management behavior is changing as the consequences for such actions become more and more severe. Coercion aside, the following are some major reasons why manufacturing employees gamble with their safety:

- *Probability*

    Risky behavior sometimes has a low probability of negative consequences. For example, if an employee understands the mechanics and functionality of a machine that he is cleaning, he can override the safety with limited risk that he will injure himself. In other words, he can ignore the safety because he believes the odds of getting hurt are in his favor.

- *Shortcuts*

    Risky behavior sometimes saves time. In manufacturing facilities, time is often very important because more time means higher levels of production...so employees resort to shortcuts. For example, an employee moving product from one area to another on the second level of storage drives her forklift with the forks five feet off the ground. She knows that, for safety reasons, she should lower the forks to the floor when moving, but she wants to save the time it takes to continually raise and lower them.

- *Simplicity*

    Risky behavior sometimes makes a job easier...and most employees want their jobs to be easier. For example, an employee overrides the safety of a production mixer so he can keep the lid open and watch product as it is mixing rather than having to stop the machine to open the lid and view the product.

Based on the above, it can be assumed that employees will behave safely if that safe behavior is easy or simple. Along the same lines, they will not behave safely if that type of behavior is difficult or challenging. Either way, the behavior becomes habit...and habits are difficult to change. Behavior based safety (also known as BBS) teaches employees about the consequences of their behavior so they develop good habits.

An important feature of BBS is that it extends beyond rank-and-file employees to supervision. It forms a safety partnership between employees and supervision where everyone watches their own behavior and that of their coworkers. It is based on management-employee relationships and is most dependent on workers trusting those in higher positions.

In a nutshell, BBS adheres to a protocol where an activator leads to behavior that produces results. The protocol is broken down as follows:

Activator

This is a condition that influences the way an employee behaves. It is the reason that an employee chooses to exhibit safe or unsafe behavior (the next part of the protocol). An example of an activator is a production employee who needs to produce a certain amount of product in order to properly do his job at a manufacturing plant.

Behavior

This is the employee's reaction to the activator. In other words, it is the action they take after being stimulated to do something. Using the activator example, the employee chooses to use safe or unsafe behavior in order to meet his production quota.

Results

These are the benefits or consequences that result from the behavior of the employee. Safe behavior is beneficial while unsafe behavior is consequential. In the activator example, unsafe behavior might cause the employee to get injured; thereby preventing him from accomplishing his production goal.

Based on the above, it can be seen that activators tell employees that they need to behave in certain ways, and results are the outcome of that behavior. In other words, activation is motivation, behavior is motivation-based action, and results are action-based consequences.

Now that you understand a little about safety and its relationship to BBS, it is time to move on to the next section that focuses on the basic principles of BBS.

Underlying Philosophy

The following are essential principles of the behavior based safety process in manufacturing:

Prevention

This might be the most important principle, and that is why is listed first. It needs to be accepted and understood by all employees that every injury, regardless of the type of seriousness, can be prevented...and safety is the key.

Along the same lines, every safety risk needs to be identified and adequately managed. "Adequately" is the key word because inadequate management does not reduce or eliminate the problem.

Management driven

In order for BBS to work properly, everyone has to be involved and take on some type of responsibility. However, management is still legally, ethically, and financially responsible for the safety of all employees in the manufacturing facility. That being said, the BBS process is management driven...and this will likely never change.

Trust

Trust is essential for the BBS process to work as designed. People need to trust each other to watch out for everyone's safety. However, this process is management driven, so most of that trust involves production employees trusting those in higher positions. This is important because once trust is lost...it is difficult to restore.

Safety is profit

If safety is viewed as an expense or cost, then the BBS system will not work properly. The prevention of injuries needs to be thought of as adding to profitability because it makes good business sense to have safe manufacturing workforces. In the long term, employee health and welfare shows up on the bottom line as black rather than red...and this makes all stakeholders happy.

Safety is paramount

Safety can never take a backseat to production. Instead, it needs to intertwine with production so each is dependent on the other to make the manufacturing facility the best that it can be. Along the same lines, safety cannot be compromised because it is more difficult than taking shortcuts. It needs to be viewed as helping an organization get better, rather than bogging it down.

Safety is not optional

All employees need to be aware from their first day of employment that they do not have a choice when it comes to safe behavior. Safety is a condition of employment, not an option that can be chosen based on discretion.

Training is necessary

All employees need training for BBS or they cannot be expected to embrace and follow the program. Education is essential, and it cannot be put on hold due to time restraints or other issues. In most workplaces training involves:

- Educating managers on how to observe and take action to prevent unsafe employee actions

- Educating employees to observe and take action to prevent their own unsafe actions
- Educating employees on how to observe and take action to prevent unsafe coworker actions
- Education managers and employees on how to take action by giving constructive feedback on their observations

Employees have safety responsibilities

It is imperative that all manufacturing employees understand their responsibilities with regard to safety. They need to make sure that their coworkers behave safely, and part of this responsibility involves stopping unsafe operations. They cannot stand by and watch their coworkers engage in unsafe behavior; they have an obligation to get involved and halt unsafe processes or procedures.

Now that you understand the thinking behind BBS in manufacturing, it is time to move into the next section that describes the BBS process as a whole.

Process

This section describes the process of BBS, and it is the crux of this book. The following are steps that need to take place in order for BBS to be successful using a manufacturing example:

Identify unsafe behavior that needs to be improved

This is more than just identifying the safety issue. It involves finding the root cause of the problem. For example, if an employee is behaving unsafely while operating a machine, then the reason for her unsafe behavior needs to be determined. It could be due to any of the following:

- She is being pushed for production quotas.
- She has not been trained and is unaware that her behavior is unsafe.
- She is told to ignore safe behavior.
- She chooses to ignore safe behavior.

Instead of telling her to "stop doing that," an understanding of the root cause needs to be determined so it can be addressed for the prevention of future safety violations.

Develop a list of ideas that can be utilized to correct the unsafe behavior

Management determines that the root cause of the employee's actions is her supervisor telling her to ignore safe behavior. Her supervisor believes the risk for injury while operating her machine is low, and safe behavior takes time that could be spent putting out higher levels of production. Based on this determination, there needs to be clarification of management's safety expectations. The list of potential corrective ideas to do this is as follows:

- Reprimand her supervisor to correct the problem and prevent a reoccurrence.

- Meet with her supervisor to correct the problem and prevent a reoccurrence.
- Meet with all supervisors to correct the problem and prevent a reoccurrence.
- Meet with all employees to correct the problem and prevent a reoccurrence.

Select the best idea from the list

Management chooses "meet with all supervisors to correct the problem and prevent a reoccurrence" as the idea they want to put into action. It is selected because supervision is the root cause of the problem, and her supervisor's behavior needs to be addressed. However, it is a known fact that all supervisors take some shortcuts and need to be made more aware of the importance of safety, so they can also benefit from the meeting.

Develop an action plan for the idea

When developing an action plan, it is important to understand that BBS uses positive reinforcement to (1) change employee behavior that is unsafe and (2) support employee behavior that is safe. Positive reinforcement differs from negative reinforcement as follows:

Positive reinforcement

Positive reinforcement increases safe behavior by focusing on non-mandatory employee efforts. In other words, it encourages workers to willingly perform above minimum standards by recognizing them for their efforts. The goal is a win-win situation where employees and the manufacturer both experience success. For example, employees who notice unsafe behavior on production lines are awarded gift certificates when they inform their supervisors.

Unfortunately, positive reinforcement does not exist in some manufacturing facilities. Employees are not recognized for their safety minded actions regardless of the effort they put forth. For example, an employee always reminds other workers to lock out machines when inspecting or cleaning them, but he never receives management praise or credit for "going the extra mile." When this happens, the employee-management relationship is minimal and trust diminishes.

Negative reinforcement

Negative reinforcement is fear based. If the employees comply, they are not disciplined...but their efforts are not recognized. The focus is on complying with a standard because compliance leads to success. This method often works to increase safety, but the only winner is the company. Employees fear repercussion for non-conformance, so they comply. For example, employees are told that they will avoid disciplinary action if they wear appropriate gloves when operating a drill press. They comply and wear the gloves to avoid punishment for not wearing them.

Some manufacturers believe only in negative reinforcement. They threaten disciplinary action for unsafe behavior, and employees comply out of fear. For example, management might threaten employees with suspension or termination if they fail to wear safety goggles while working on a lathe. This causes the employee-management relationship to deteriorate quickly...and employees lose trust in their bosses.

As noted earlier, the action plan is to have a meeting with supervisors to discuss the problem. In this meeting, management explains the safety issues that they have observed, and they explain why this behavior is unsafe. They share their ideas for change and ask for suggestions in order to create a safer manufacturing process and prevent future safety problems from occurring. Once an agreement is reached, it is time for the implementation phase.

Implement the action plan

This is where ideas become reality. At the manufacturing facility, all supervisors meet with their employees to explain the new safety policies, protocols, and procedures. They offer training to any employee who would like to go through it, and they express confidence that their employees will perform their jobs with safety as a top priority.

Evaluate the success of the action plan

The changes made to the manufacturing facility need to be monitored for success. This is done when management directly observes employee safety behavior and reviews documented safety violations and work-related injuries. When employees perform their jobs safely, they receive feedback in the form of praise or rewards. This is an important part of the BBS process because it assures the plan is effective and continues to work as expected using positive reinforcement as a motivator.

Now let's examine a complete example that can be used as a model for manufacturers. The BBS process below was implemented in a paper towel manufacturing plant. It has real-world application and can be used as a model for building other BBS programs.

Wilson Paper Supply
Behavior Based Safety Process

Scope

Wilson Paper Supply (as known as the company) is a paper towel manufacturing plant located in Chicago, IL. The company employs 250 people including 190 production employees. Nick VanDeer is employed as the company's safety manager and oversees all safety related operations, including a safety team that consists of the plant manager, the quality control manager, and the office manager. The safety team meets once per month to discuss safety concerns in the facility.

Safety problem

The safety team has identified forklift driving in the warehouse as unsafe behavior that needs to be improved. There have not been any documented injuries, but employees have complained to management on three separate occasions that forklift drivers are exhibiting unsafe behavior. It appears that it is only a matter of time before someone gets hurt.

Specific issues with forklift drivers include:

- They sometimes fail to yield for employees walking through the warehouse.
- They sometimes drive forklifts at unsafe speeds.
- They sometimes drive outside the yellow lines that they are instructed to stay within.

Root cause

After interviewing the forklift drivers, the team has determined that the problem is not due to lack of knowledge or misunderstanding. The drivers understand the rules, but they have limited time to get their work done and subsequently do not always follow them.

Potential solutions

The following are potential solutions for correcting the forklift driver's unsafe behavior:

- Terminate the drivers who have exhibited unsafe behavior.
- Threaten to suspend forklift drivers who violate safety rules.
- Meet with the forklift driver's to discuss their unsafe behavior.
- Meet with other managers to discuss the forklift driver's unsafe behavior.
- Meet with all employees to discuss the forklift driver's unsafe behavior.

Chosen solution

The team decides to meet with the forklift drivers to discuss their unsafe behavior. This gives the safety team an opportunity to explain the reasoning behind the rules, and it allows the drivers to ask questions or request clarification. Management and the other employees are not needed in this meeting because the drivers' individual behavior is the specific issue that needs to be addressed.

Action plan

Upon meeting with the drivers, Nick VanDeer (safety team leader) starts by explaining to the forklift drivers that some employees have expressed concerns to management about unsafe forklift driving. Nick describes the mentioned driver actions below and explains why they are unsafe.

- *The drivers sometimes fail to yield for employees walking through the warehouse*

Employees often need to cross over forklift paths, so management has designated specific crossing areas. Management realizes the time is important at the paper towel manufacturing plant and drivers want to be efficient at their jobs...but employees should not have to fear accidents when crossing at designated areas.

- *The drivers sometimes drive forklifts at unsafe speeds*

  Employees work alongside forklift drivers in some areas of the plant, so management has posted yellow "SLOW" signs in those areas. Again, management realizes that time is important because drivers want to optimize their performance, but employees should not have to worry about being hit by a forklift that is going too fast to stop in time.

- *The drivers sometimes drive outside the yellow lines that they are instructed to stay within*

  Employees need to move around to different areas of the plant, so management has drawn yellow lines on the floor to separate forklift paths and employees. Management realizes that it virtually impossible to stay within the yellow lines 100 percent of the time, but employees should not have to fear getting hit by forklifts when they are in their designated areas.

After explaining the safety issues, Nick asks the drivers for suggestions on what could be done to create a safer work environment. One driver suggests that the shipping manager should stop pushing them so hard to get their work done. Nick agrees this is a good idea, but he says that this is not the shipping manager's fault because he is being pressured by the salespeople to fill last minute orders. However, he can initiate some changes to prevent this from happing on a regular basis. Another driver suggests an incentive program where drivers are rewarded for safe behavior. Nick says safe behavior is expected by all employees, but he can come up with something to help them in this area.

The meeting adjourns, and Nick promises to get back with the drivers the next day with potential resolutions to the problem.

The following day, the safety team again meets with the drivers. Nick proposes the following solutions:

- *Salespeople will be required to put in their order one day before they need to be filled.*

  The sales manager will meet with all salespeople and explain to them that safety is a top priority, and rush orders are creating an unsafe work environment. Understandably, this is not always possible...but it is definitely an area that can and will be improved.

- *Drivers will earn one extra vacation day for every four months that they go without an accident or a complaint.*

This means the drivers have an opportunity to earn three paid vacation days per year for practicing safe behavior based on written documentation and evaluation by their coworkers.

The drivers agree with Nick's proposal, and the action plan goes into effect at the start of the next work week. Nick expresses confidence in the forklift drivers' ability to be successful, and he tells the drivers that he will share the results with them via an email to their manager at the end of each month.

Evaluation

One year after the BBS process has been implemented, the results are analyzed and it is found that the process is successful. Forklift drivers are practicing safe behavior, and this is verified by the following:

- *Ongoing discussion with plant employees has yielded no complaints since the BBS process was implemented.*

- *All drivers have been awarded at least two vacation days since the BBS process was implemented.*

- *Tracking of sales data indicates rush orders are down 75 percent since the BBS process was implemented.*

Follow-up

For the next two years, the safety team meets every six months to discuss forklift driver safety. They review sales data and employee complaints regarding forklift driver safety. Additionally, they have one forklift driver and two plant employees attend the meeting to voluntary discuss the ongoing success of the BBS process. After each meeting, positive feedback is given about the success that is continually being experienced.

Benefits

There are many benefits that stem from BBS. Some of these benefits documented, such as reduced work-related injuries, while some are not documented, such as improvement of employees' attitudes.

The following are all positives that result from BBS:

- *Elimination of current practices of unsafe behavior*

   This is the major reason for the implementation of BBS. Once up and running, BBS eliminates existing unsafe behavior and replaces it with safe practices.

- *Prevention of future unsafe behavior*

BBS puts safety first. Safety does not take a backseat to production in manufacturing plants, and this means it is at the top of every employee's agenda. The workers' mindsets prevent them from taking safety risks; thereby preventing unsafe behavior in the future.

- *Reduced documented injuries*

  This benefit is documented. When safety is at the forefront, unsafe behavior decreases....and so do workplace injuries. This is one of management's favorite benefits because the reduction is quantifiable.

- *Reduced OSHA intervention*

  Fewer workplace injuries lead to fewer visits from OSHA officials. This means OSHA violations are reduced...as are the cost of their fines. This is also high on the list of favorite benefits for management because it equates to fewer headaches and expenses...especially in manufacturing facilities.

- *Increased morale*

  Rewards and positive reinforcement are both a part of successful BBS processes. People's morale is raised when they are acknowledged for their good actions, and that acknowledgment comes from rewards. Positive reinforcement also raises employees' morale; thereby making them more likely to perform at peak levels.

- *Avoidance of the "blame-game"*

  BBS does not place blame on any one individual. The goal is to improve safety as a whole by making everyone aware of unsafe behavior. Rather than place blame on their coworkers, employees watch out for each other creating a win-win situation for the company and the people employed by it.

- *Open two-way communication*

  BBS is all about management-employee communication regarding safety. This opens the door for candid discussion about other issues; thereby creating an environment of open two-way communication.

The above benefits of BBS show that the system is worth implementing. However, as might be expected, there are also some negatives associated with this concept. The following section focuses on the challenges involved with BBS.

Challenges

If you ask critics, they will tell you that there are many challenges associated with BBS. In fact, all one needs to do is search the Internet, and they will find their share of negative comments. The scope of this book does not allow for listing all of those comments, but it does extract four major criticisms as follows:

- *Employees are rewarded for not reporting unsafe behavior*

  BBS has been accused of creating a very contradictory situation because it rewards employees for not reporting unsafe behavior. For example, if production workers know that they will receive a bonus for plant-wide reduced injuries, then they will not report certain injuries. In other words, the BBS system ends up doing what it was supposed to prevent. The injuries are still there, but they are covered up because employees would rather have the added compensation.

- *Unsafe behavior is not always the cause of injuries*

  Many manufacturing plants have old or poorly maintained machines in operation. These machines break down regularly; thereby creating unsafe situations that have nothing to do with employee behavior. Regardless of their safety practices, employees get injured due to circumstances that are out of their control.

  It might seem like a simple fix to this problem is to invest in new machinery. Yes, that works, but it is often easier said than done. Some manufacturers simply do not have the money to invest so they keep the old machinery operational for periods of time that far exceed normal expectations. If this is the situation, then BBS is nothing more than a grand illusion.

- *Supervisor limits*

  Most organizations that implement BBS expect supervisors to do more work in terms of safety observation. In theory, this sounds great...but it is often not realistic. Manufacturing supervisors are increasingly expected to do more with fewer resources, and their time needs to be spent on other important issues. In short, supervisors do not have the capacity to operate BBS processes as intended....so the processes ultimately fail.

- *Union opposition*

  Some unions strongly oppose BBS because they believe the process encourages employees to get into conflicts and disagreements about safety. It is not a production worker's job to tell another production employee that they need to change their unsafe behavior. Union employees are supposed to unite and work together, not "rat-out" each other and become quarrelsome.

  Some unions also believe that management tends to see BBS as "cure-all" that absolves them of their own safety responsibility. They simply pass that responsibility on to their employees, and the employees argue among themselves until they find a resolution.

Finally, some unions believe managers see BBS as a way to save money in their departments. Rather than spend money to fix equipment and machines, they spend time changing employees' unsafe behavior. This might work for a short period of time, but it ultimately ends up making manufacturing workplaces more unsafe.

Summary

Behavior based safety is a process that works to eliminate and prevent unsafe behavior. It uses positive reinforcement by rewarding employees who perform above minimum standards; thereby benefiting workers and the organizations that employ them.

This book focuses on behavior based safety in manufacturing. It introduces the topic, discusses its underlying principles, and provides a real-world example that can be used as a model for manufacturing facilities. The text is informational and educational, and it is written for easy reader application and understanding.

Congratulations! You now understand more about behavior based safety...an important aspect of many manufacturing operations.

Employee Safety and Building Security

An Introduction to Worker and Workplace Protection

Louis Bevoc

Published by
NutriNiche System LLC

Louis Bevoc books...simple explanations of complex subjects

Summary

Introduction

Employee safety and building security are much more prevalent topics that they were in the not so distant past. This is because unsafe working conditions are now a concern for many organizations. These conditions occur for a variety of reasons including arguments, disputes, affairs, termination, mental illness, differences in beliefs, and perceived wrongful treatment. However, regardless of the reasons why unsafe conditions occur, the consequences are severe and sometimes even deadly. Based on this reality, it is important that workplaces are as safe and secure as possible to protect employees from potential harm.

Please consider the following in regard to employee safety and building security:

Importance of employee safety

Every employee has the right to be employed in a workplace that is safe. They should not have to worry about being robbed, attacked, or physically assaulted in any way, and there are laws to enforce this protection. However, aside from the legal aspects involved, leaders of organizations should be concerned about worker safety for the following reasons:

Perception

Unsafe workplaces create poor perceptions of organizations. That perception comes from employees, suppliers, customers, regulatory agencies, and the public.

Employees who believe a workplace is unsafe can put the word out that it is not a good place to work. They deter their friends, family, and acquaintances from becoming employees, and this causes organizations to lose out on potentially good workers.

OSHA, a government safety watchdog, hits unsafe organizations hard. They levy fines for violations, and they go after repeat offenders. Organizations that are perceived as unsafe can expect a visit from OSHA...especially if an employee "blows the whistle."

Customers who perceive organizations as unsafe might choose not to purchase their products or services. Lost sales can be detrimental to organizations...even causing them to go out of business.

Suppliers might choose not to sell to organizations they perceive as unsafe for ethical reasons. In this respect, they are risking the well-being of their own organization because principle is more important than profitability.

Public opinion is likely the most damaging type of perception. People boycott organizations they perceive as unsafe, and that results in lost sales that are critical for survival. The worst thing about poor public perception is the fact that it can be very difficult to change.

Profitability

Money talks. In fact, sometimes money is the only reason that leaders or organizations listen...simply because their jobs are threatened. When organizations are not safe, they cost those leaders money in the form of lawsuits.

Sexual harassment is a good example of unsafe working conditions that lead to lawsuits. People feel unsafe around a coworker due to his or her sexual advances, and they want to be compensated for the fear they are experiencing.

Another cost that leads to lower profits is absenteeism. When employees do not feel safe, they do not show up for work. When they are absent, their jobs suffer...and this impacts the bottom lines of organizations.

Productivity

Unsafe work environments lead to injury or illness. Injury is physical, such as getting hurt while working on a machine. Illness, however, can be physical or mental. Physical illness results from exposure to harmful aspects of the workplace, such as working in an environment where toxic vapors are not properly exhausted.   Mental illness results from the stress of working in an unsafe environment, as is the case when employees are so worried about unsafe aspects of their jobs that they are unable to come to work.

As might be expected, workplace productivity diminishes for employees who are ill or injured. They also lose trust in management, and that trust is difficult to get back once it is lost.

Preservation

This refers to preservation of the workforce. In other words, preservation means minimizing turnover by retaining employees. Workers who do not feel safe at their jobs will look for other employment...and the turnover can be devastating. In fact, as some people have experienced, severe cases of turnover stop organizations from functioning.

Importance of building security

Secure buildings do not guarantee that the employees inside will be safe. However, building security does prevent many external threats from entering the facility, thereby lowering safety risks for employees inside. It also prevents unsafe activity outside the physical structure by monitoring the building and grounds.

Building security is important for the following reasons:

Deterrence

If there are efforts in place to secure a building, unauthorized people will think twice about entering it. The security in place deters behavior or activity that will lead to the safety concerns for the people inside or outside the building.

Theft

Unfortunately, theft in organizations is not rare. In certain small ways, all employees unconsciously take things that are not theirs...such as going home with pens or pencils.   However, this discussion is concerned with conscious theft that results in people feeling violated.

Common items stolen internally include money, cell phones, computers, office supplies, small equipment, and machine parts. Common items stolen externally include vehicles, vehicle parts, stored equipment, and valuable parts of the building itself.

Theft inside and outside of organizations is something that likely never be eliminated. However, building security is a good way to reduce occurrences. Simple monitoring of the building and grounds alert the security personnel to dishonest behavior.

Vandalism

Vandalism refers to the destruction of company or personal property. Typically, external vandalism involves destruction of the building, grounds, or vehicles (personal and company). Internal vandalism involves equipment, supplies, fixtures, and personal belongings.

When employees witnessed vandalism, they often feel unsafe because they fear what might happen next. They are not sure if the destruction will lead to attacks or other violent acts, so they fear for their own safety.

Evidence

If a picture is worth a thousand words, then a video is worth a million words. Nothing tells the truth better than a video because it is an undisputable fact. Video provides information that identifies activities that make workplaces unsafe.

Employees might not like the fact that they are always on camera, but they can take comfort in the fact that those cameras provide a service in troubling situations. Video provides evidence of what transpired, and this evidence helps workplaces maintain safety and security.

This book focuses on employee safety and building security. More specifically, it examines ways in which organizations can be made more safe and secure for the workers employed by them. First, it discusses external and internal lines of defense, next it examines management and human resources' responsibilities, and then it suggests ways to improve safety and security programs. The text is informational and educational, and it is written for easy reader understanding at all levels.

Now that you understand the scope of this book and have been introduced to the subject matter, let's move into external lines of defense that organizations have in place.

External Lines of Defense

This refers to the line of protection that an organization has in place outside of the building where the employees work. It is often the most complex and well-thought defense system because it keeps people from entering the facility where they can create unsafe working conditions.

Essentially, an external line of defense has four major goals. These goals are below, and they are listed in order of importance for the strongest protection.

- *Discourage unsafe activity*

    As the saying goes, "an ounce of prevention is worth a pound of cure." This is very true for external lines of defense, and that is why the discouraging of unsafe activity is the first and foremost goal. If unsafe activity can be prevented, then the building and grounds will remain safe.

    An example of discouraging unsafe activity is a high fence around the parking lot of a manufacturing plant. Thieves looking to break into or steal vehicles know they have to penetrate the fence to get to the vehicles, and this deters them from moving forward with their devious plans of action. The external line of defense works to keep the parking lot safe.

- *Perceive unsafe activity*

    If something is suspicious, notice it immediately. Abrupt awareness is critical because it allows time for analyzing the unsafe situation and preparing a potential plan of action.

    An example is a white van that drives by a bank three times. An alert security guard becomes suspicious, so she writes down a description of the van, the occupants, and a license plate number. She wants to be sure that she has this information available if there is an attempt to rob the bank or any of its customers.

- *Stop unsafe activity*

    If suspicious behavior or activity turns into reality, then put a stop to it as soon as possible. Plans should be in place to end safety problems before they fester into bigger concerns.

An example is a security guard who witnesses a lunchtime fight break out between two employees at a picnic table outside the building. He immediately moves in to break up the fight and then documents the incident by taking statements from each employee and all witnesses.

- *Report unsafe activity*

    Unfortunately, some activity cannot be stopped. If this is the case, then it must be reported to the proper authorities. These authorities include the local police and management of the organization.

    An example is a security guard who witnesses an employee getting robbed by two assailants while walking to his vehicle after work. The robbers flee in a car before the security guard can reach them, so she immediately calls the police and reports the suspects fled in a blue Chevy Caprice going north on Main Street. After she calls the police, she calls the general manager of the organization where she is employed to inform him of the incident.

Unsafe activity comes in many different forms, and it needs to be combatted before it has a chance to enter the building and cause more damage. Based on this, external lines of defense must always try to get better... so the above goals should be part of a continuous improvement process.

The following are some suggestions for helping achieve continuous improvement of external defense programs:

Fencing

Fencing can surround the parking lot, building, or entire property of an organization. It typically ranges in height from four feet to ten feet and sometimes has barbed wire at the top of it. In extreme cases, fencing is electrified to deter people with harmful intent. Regardless of the physical makeup, fencing is a very effective barrier for keeping unsafe activity outside of designated areas.

Gates

Gates are often used as the only entrance point for fenced areas. Some gates only allow employees, vendors, suppliers, salespeople, regulatory agencies inside, while others are big enough for vehicles to enter. Regardless of the gate size, they work well for monitoring anyone or anything that comes into a designated area.

Gate passes often accompany gates. These are given to authorized personnel to enter the gated areas. They allow for fast access and do not require a guard to be present, but guards are still necessary for unauthorized personnel. They ask people for identification and the reason for their visit. Gates are a great way to improve external lines of defense, but they require guards to be completely effective.

Patrol guards

These guards are not confined to a particular station, such as a gate entrance. Instead, they roam the premises looking for issues that might lead to unsafe situations. They travel by vehicle or on foot, but the idea is to continually monitor the grounds for suspicious or unsafe activity.

Limited entrances

This refers to the building itself. Many companies have designated entrances for employees and visitors with different protocols for each after someone enters the facility. Unauthorized people raise a red flag when they enter through the wrong door, and this helps minimize unsafe activity.

Lighting

It is very difficult to see outdoor activity at night if there is no light. Night vision equipment negates the need for light, but most organizations do not have it or cannot afford it. Not surprisingly, unsafe activity increases in darkness, and that is why adequate outdoor lighting is critical for organizations. This lighting should shine on the building and the premises to deter potential unsafe activity, and it should be sufficient to detect activity in all hiding places.

Cameras

Most people understand the importance of cameras. These devices document behavior and activities and lead to the resolution of many problems. As might be expected, cameras are an excellent tool for detecting unsafe behavior...and that is why they help organizations achieve continuous improvement in the area of safety.

Telephone hotlines

Telephone hotlines have been a part of college campuses and hospitals for some time now, but the concept also has application in other organizations looking to improve safety and security. All people have to do is pick up a conveniently located phone to report suspicious activity and the appropriate people will respond. In this regard, everyone acts as a security guard and unsafe activity is minimized.

Open space

Essentially, this refers to reducing hiding areas. Equipment storage, unused vehicles, clutter, and debris all provide the potential spots where wrongdoers can remain undetected while conducting unsafe activities. Open space is necessary for seeing everything that is happening, and that is why it is an important part of continuously improving an external line of defense.

Now you are aware of external lines of defense and methods for helping them continuously improve. Unfortunately, an external line of defense will not prevent all unsafe activity. Some problems get past external defenses and enter the building while others begin inside the facility. This leads us to the next section that discusses preventing and controlling unsafe activity inside buildings...better known as internal lines of defense.

Internal lines of defense

The following are reasons why internal lines of defense are necessary to combat unsafe activity:

- The external line of defense functioned as designed, but it was not enough to prevent the unsafe activity from entering the facility.

  An example is an employee who hides a gun under his coat with the intent of shooting a coworker. External security recognizes the employee, but cannot see the hidden gun. They allow the employee to enter the building because this is normal protocol.

- The external line of defense did not function as designed, and an error allowed the unsafe activity to enter the building.

  An example is a person who lies to the gate guard that she is a salesperson who has a meeting with a purchasing agent. She is actually there to confront a supervisor who fired her husband, but the guard does not ask any further questions and allows her past the gate where she can enter the building.

- The external line of defense could not prevent the unsafe activity because that activity began inside the facility.

  An example is an employee who overrides a safety on a machine to get his job done faster. External lines of defense cannot prevent this from happening because the unsafe activity was never outside the building.

Internal lines of defense have the same major goals as external lines, but internal situations are more serious because the unsafe activity has entered the building. These goals are below, and they are listed in order of importance for the strongest protection.

- *Discourage unsafe activity*

  The unsafe activity is in the building, but it can be prevented from penetrating further into the facility and causing more damage.

  For example, a person with a hidden gun might get through the exterior line of defense and enter the building. However, after seeing the metal detector, he changes his mind and leaves because he realizes his hidden weapon will be discovered.

- *Perceive unsafe activity*

  If something is suspicious, notice it immediately. Abrupt awareness is critical because it allows time for analyzing the situation and preparing a potential plan of action.

An example office clerk who overhears an employee tell a coworker that he is going to "beat his boss to a pulp" for writing him up for attendance issues. The office clerk immediately tells her supervisor, who informs the general manager and security at the organization.

- ## *Stop unsafe activity*

If suspicious behavior or activity turns into reality, then put a stop to it as soon as possible. Plans should be in place to end safety problems before they fester into bigger concerns.

An example is horseplay in a production area. One employee is pulling another on the forks of an electric jack. The employees think this situation is funny, but the shipping manager views it as dangerous where someone could get hurt. The shipping manager puts an immediate stop to this unsafe activity and warns the employees that their actions will be documented.

- ## *Report unsafe activity*

Unfortunately, some activity cannot be stopped. If this is the case, then it must be reported to the proper authorities. These authorities include the local police and management of the organization.

An example is a supervisor who hears one of his employees threaten to kill another employee over a dispute. The threat has already been made so it cannot be stopped. However, based on the unsafe work environment created by the offending employee, the supervisor reports the incident to management and the local police.

A plan of actions must be in effect as soon as the unsafe activity enters the building...typically at the front desk or in a lobby. Like external lines of defense, internal lines of defense also need continuous improvement.

The following are tools that can be utilized for continuously improving internal lines of defense include:

Guards

Security guards are employed inside facilities of many different types of organizations to assure workplaces are safe. They are usually found at the main entrance or lobby where they examine people and ask questions before allowing them to enter the building. However, some security guards also patrol the entire facility. They roam from place to place looking for suspicious activity that might result in an unsafe work environment.

Metal detection

This check finds metal objects, such as guns and knives, which are known to create unsafe workplace situations. It is likely the best tool for finding dangerous objects that people are hiding. Metal detection is a fairly common part of internal lines of defense in government agencies and airports, and many companies are starting to follow suit.

Physical searches

Physical searches find objects that metal detection is not capable of discovering. Bags, purses, briefcases, satchels, boxes, and containers brought in by people are searched for things that could make workplaces unsafe. Examples include poisonous chemicals, liquid explosives, bats, and clubs. These types of searches are quite common at large scale sporting events and concerts.

Body scans

These devices use radio waves to scan people's entire bodies for potentially unsafe objects. They negate the need for metal detection and physical searches, but they are very uncommon due to the cost involved. Body scans are typically used by airports because hijacking has made the safety of passengers on board a major concern.

ID tags

The purpose of these tags is to identify people in order to help determine their purpose for being in the building. ID tags also indicate the people wearing them have gone through some type of security check before they were allowed to enter the building, and this creates a sense of safety for employees.

Escorts

People who are designated to accompany visitors in a facility are known as escorts. Escorts provide assurance that the visitors will not engage in activities that lead to unsafe workplace situations.

Now you are aware of internal lines of defense in organizations and way for improving them. This leads us to the role that management plays in making sure employees are safe and buildings are secure.

Management responsibilities

Employee safety and building security, like many other aspects of organizations, starts at the top. In other words, it starts with management and works its way down to rank and file employees. That being said, management needs to develop a safety and security program, assign responsibility, monitor activity, evaluate performance, and make changes for continuous improvement.

Development of the program begins with a plan. This plan must (1) define the goals of the safety and security program and (2) develop a strategy that accomplishes those goals. Management needs to formulate the plan, and then it is followed through and supported by lower level employees.

Much of the strategy involves rules and regulations. What type of external and internal line of defense will be used? What is considered unsafe activity? What is the protocol when unsafe activity is detected? No plan is foolproof, but there needs to be established structure and order. Situations that fall outside of the designated guidelines need to be dealt with on a case-by-case basis.

As the plan progresses, it becomes more detailed. Specific roles of employees need to be defined, and responsibility needs to be assigned. Will a contracted service be retained or will company employees be involved? What will the designated individuals do? Who will ultimately be responsible for the program? These are important questions, and management needs to provide the answers.

Once roles have been defined, the plan can be implemented. Responsible personnel begin to monitor the environment looking for unsafe behavior. This monitoring includes:

- Understanding who should be on the premises at all times and the type of information that is necessary to identify these people. For example, security guards at gates and entrances should make sure employees have identification, name tags, badges or uniforms...something that tells who they are and why they are on the property. Visitors should provide the names of the people they are there to see, and those people should be contacted to validate the legitimacy of the meetings. Contractors should show identification and state the work that they are performing. In the case of contractors, there should be a list of ongoing activities at the organization that can be referenced for verification of all contractor claims.

  Once people have been identified and determined to be legitimately on the premises, there should be an understanding of their areas of access. For example, the general manager has access to anywhere in the facility, but salespeople only allowed in the department of the people they are calling on. Additionally, salespeople should only be at the building during normal business hours, but the general manager can be there at any time.

- Watching for odd or unusual behavior that appears suspicious. For example, an hourly production employee who comes in carrying two briefcases arouses suspicion. This individual does not have an office job, and two briefcases are certainly not required for assembling products on a line.

  Worker start and finish times can also throw up a red flag. Employees who work on first shift should have a good reason for being on the grounds at 1:00 am. Along the same lines, people who start working at 4:00 pm should have a legitimate reason for being on the property at 10:00 am.

  Other skeptical activity includes inquiry from non-employees. Questions that should arouse suspicion include:

  > When does the second shift end?
  > What time does the supervisor usually leave?
  > How many people are in the building at midnight?
  > What time do employees arrive in the morning?

  Individuals who ask these questions are looking to gather information that should not be divulged for safety purposes.

- Observing mental and physical health or condition of people on the grounds. Employees who appear fatigued or physically ill might present a safety threat to themselves or their coworkers on the job. Sick people might have contagious diseases that could be spread through the workforce. More importantly, people experiencing high levels of stress or mental health issues are a concern because their behavior is unpredictable.

  Regardless of the type of health concern, people involved with safety and security programs need to be aware that mental and physical health issues could result in safety and security issues. This awareness can prevent problems...and possibly even save people's lives.

- Watching the non-human element. People are not the only concern in terms of employee safety and building security. Many different types of materials and supplies enter and leave the premises of organizations every day, and these can ultimately cause work environments to become unsafe. For this reason, materials and supplies also need to be monitored by the responsible personnel.

  Poisonous or toxic chemicals are a good example of materials that pose safety risks. Industrial manufacturers are the biggest concern here because they bring in a wide variety of potentially lethal chemicals, but most organizations use some chemicals for heating, refrigeration, cleaning, and pest control. If those chemicals are used improperly or end up in the wrong hands, then the result can be devastating. Think about poisonous chemicals ending up in food products that get distributed regionally or nationally, and it is rather easy to visualize the harm that can be done.

  Trucks delivering materials and suppliers should be inspected with a generic checklist. Labels should be examined and purchase orders should match up with delivery paperwork. A little vigilance can go a long way in terms of safety and security.

- Watching package and mail delivery. Delivery personnel should be uniform and be driving an official or company vehicle.   If this is not the case, then the drivers should be asked for identification to prove who they are and where they work. Sometimes this is so important that organizations have all mail and packages go through metal detectors and x-ray before reaching the intended personnel.

- Observing activity around public utilities. One often overlooked area that needs to be monitored is utilities because damage or tampering can easily lead to unsafe situations. Contaminated water can cause people to become ill, leaking gas lines can cause headaches and unconsciousness, and power outages cause darkness that can result in injuries. This means water hydrants, gas lines, and electrical transformers need to be continuously monitored. Again, a little bit of observation can prevent serious safety and security issues.

Findings from any type of monitoring activities need to be reported to management for evaluation of the overall safety and security program. If the program is working to keep employees safe and buildings secure, then it should continue with no changes. However, if problems or weaknesses are detected, then the plan needs to be reassessed so changes can be made.

Regardless of the findings, management should reassess the safety and security program on an annual basis. Reassessment makes sure the program is doing what it is intended to do. Shortcomings and weaknesses are brought to the forefront so the necessary modifications can be made. Reassessment exposes previously undetected problems that need to be addressed....and this is good for the organization and the people that work in it.

Now that you understand the significance of management in safety and security programs, let's move on to the next section that discusses the role that human resources personnel have in this process.

Human Resources' responsibilities

Good management is critical for making sure employees are safe and buildings are secure. However, human resource departments also play an important role in the process as follows:

Hiring

This is the most important role that human resources personnel play because, if done correctly, it stops people who create safety issues from becoming employees. To weed out problem employees, human resources personnel need to conduct background checks on everyone before hiring them. These checks can find out a lot of information about individuals...including their history of unsafe behavior at previous jobs.

Three major checks that need to be conducted include:

Criminal history

This indicates past crimes committed, but, more importantly, it shows any type of problematic behavior that might be related to workplace safety issues.

Employer history

This indicates things an employee might have done are not typically mentioned on a resume or during an interview. For obvious reasons, past unsafe behavior is not something that most people willingly divulge.

Academic history

Academic history is important because unsafe behavior by universities or colleges is often a permanent part of a student's file. Again, this is something that most people do not want a potential employer to know.

Training

This refers to the training the people responsible for employee safety and building security go through. It shows personnel how to detect and respond to actions that can threaten safety at workplaces. It also demonstrates, through lecture and example, the importance of safety and security so the responsible employees take their jobs more seriously.

Training can be expensive, but it is well worth the cost if done correctly. It should start with an orientation and be an ongoing part of the process in order to introduce new ideas and concepts.

In short, training should:

- Make responsible employees aware that there is no tolerance for unsafe activity. Any unsafe activity will be dealt with swiftly, and the punishment might include termination from the organization.

- Encourage responsible employees to report all unsafe behavior to those in charge. Those employees must know that their reporting will be taken seriously and followed up on.

- Help responsible employees understand the need for the perception of a safe and secure environment. This helps deter unsafe behavior by making people think twice about their actions.

- Show responsible employees how to listen to people's concerns and act accordingly. Their involvement is critical for stopping unsafe behavior and preventing it from festering in the workplace.

Improving

Employee security and safety programs need to constantly strive to get better. In other words, management should always be looking for improvement. Some suggestions for improving these programs include:

- *Intensify background checks*

  It has been said that there can never be enough background checks on potential employees. While this might be a bit overboard, the point is well taken. Leaders of organizations should intensify the background checks of potential personnel for the protection of their business and employees. This can be done by strengthening existing programs using online background check services, or professional firms that specialize in this area can be hired. Either way, information can be gathered to keep workplaces safe and secure.

- *Utilize local authorities*

  This is likely the most unknown way to improve safety and security programs. Many local organizations, such as the police, firefighters, and OSHA, will come to facilities to provide information or train personnel. They will also conduct safety assessments that identify areas of weakness and make management aware of areas where they need to improve.

  Local authorities want to help organizations become safer because it helps make their jobs easier in the long run. Reach out to them, and they will respond accordingly.

- *Contract professional organizations*

Workplaces can be made safer by hiring outside firms to handle all security issues. These companies employ professionals who are trained to identify, stop, and prevent unsafe activities in and around the buildings where people work. They also understand exactly what is required for the best external and internal lines of defense, thereby preventing unsafe behavior from penetrating into the building where it can do further damage.

Professional organizations take care of security needs and the headaches that go along with them….and this makes them well worth the cost.

- *Utilize technology*

Every organization is different, but they all have safety and security needs. Those needs can be addressed with technology that makes employers and employees feel safer in their work environment.

This is the age of technology, and organizations need to take advantage of it. Leaders of workplaces can no longer use cost as a reason to ignore technological advances because many of those advances are very realistically priced. Camera systems, computer software programs, specialized lighting, and metal detection are all options that should be explored to improve employee safety and building security.

- *Rehearse*

Employees involved in safety and security programs need to be able to act quickly and effectively to problems and emergencies, and they are best prepared for this using practice drills and role-playing exercises. These types of activities force people to react and make decisions in challenging situations that they may encounter in their jobs.

Practice drills and role-playing exercises are often disdained because they do not seem realistic and take people out of their comfort zones… but they do have some benefits for safety training. They build confidence because employees get to experience a wide variety of different safety scenarios. They also develop problem-solving skills because workers need to think about situations in order to come up with potential solutions.

Rehearsal for real situations is something that is gaining attention in organizations worldwide. There has been success with this concept…and it can help prevent safety issues in workplaces.

- *Implement written policies*

This is the easiest way to improve safety and security programs because any organization can implement policies. Policies set a clear tone of what is expected of employees. They promote positive behavior and outline discipline protocols for violating established rules.

These policies must be written, and they can be distributed to employees in a variety of ways. They can be handed out, emailed, or posted on employee bulletin boards. However, the best and most effective way to introduce them is during employee training or meetings. Employee signatures indicate they understand the rules involving safety and security in the workplace, and signatures are difficult to dispute when problems occur. This assures management that discipline can be taken without fear of future legal action.

Summary

Employee safety and building security are more important today than they have ever been in the past. People want to feel safe in and around the organizations that employ them, but a variety of different factors prevent them from experiencing that feeling. Because of this, workplace leaders must invest time and resources into the protection of their people and property.

This book focuses on employee safety and building security. First, it examines external and internal lines of defense that organizations utilize. Next, it explores the role of management and the support that human resources departments provide. Then it suggests ways for improving safety and security processes. The text is informational and educational, and it is written for easy reader understanding at all levels.

Congratulations! You now understand more about employee safety and building security.... high priority concerns for workers all over the world.

Reference Handbook of Safety Risks in Manufacturing
12 Important Concerns and Why They Exist

Louis Bevoc

Published by
NutriNiche System LLC

Louis Bevoc books...simple explanations of complex subjects

Introduction

Introduction

This book is about safety risks in manufacturing facilities. It would not be complete without an introduction to The Occupational Safety and Health Administration (also known as OSHA)...so this is where it begins. OSHA was formed by the United States government in 1971 to assure the safety of workers in American. Like most government agencies, it has grown in size over the years and presently employs over 2000 people with an annual budget that exceed 500 million dollars.

OSHA protects most private sector employees and certain public sector workers in the 50 states. It also has jurisdiction in the Virgin Islands, Guam, Puerto Rico, and the District of Columbia. Individually tailored safety and health plans operate in over 20 states, but these plans are approved, funded, and monitored by OSHA. OSHA directly covers certain workplaces excluded from state plans such as military bases and maritime industries. Essentially, the only people not covered by some form of OSHA are self-employed farm employees and their immediate families...but these individuals are regulated by other federal agencies.

OSHA law states that all employers must comply with specific rules and regulations and have workplaces that do not contain serious safety or health hazards. The law also requires employers to seek out and correct serious health and safety issues without relying solely on personal protective equipment (gloves, goggles, boots, shields, etc.). For example, a barrier should be put around a machine with a hot surface rather than relying on gloves that protect employees if they come in contact with that surface.

Other requirements of OSHA include the following:

- Temporary employees must be treated the same as permanent employees in terms of health and safety. They are not excluded from OSHA rules and regulations simply because they are not employees of the workplace where they are performing their jobs.
- Employees have the right to work in environments that do not pose serious health and safety risks including workplaces with high noise levels.
- Personal protective equipment (PPE) must be provided to all employees who need it, and it must be provided to those employees at no cost.
- Health and safety training must be conducted in a manner that is understood by the entire workforce, and language and literacy barriers must be overcome.
- OSHA must be notified of all work-related in-patient hospitalizations, amputations, and losses of an eye within 24 hours of the occurrence, and OHSA must be notified of all work-related fatalities within 8 hours of the occurrence.
- OSHA rights and responsibilities posters must be displayed for viewing by all employees.
- All OSHA citations must be documented and displayed for viewing by all employees.
- Work-related injuries and illnesses must be documented and displayed for viewing by all employees.

Additionally:

- Employees have the right to report workplace health and safety concerns or ask for an inspection of their workplace, and employers are not allowed to retaliate against them for these actions. Employees who are retaliated against for their actions have the right to file a complaint with OSHA under the Whistleblower Act. The Whistleblower Act is specifically designed to prevent employees from being afraid to speak up about workplace concerns.
- Employees have the right to ask for and receive records of all workplace injuries and illnesses.

- Employees have the right to participate in OSHA inspections, ask questions, and speak to OSHA inspectors privately.

If OSHA inspectors find violations during a workplace audit, they are authorized to issue citations and penalize the employer monetarily in the form of fines...with the maximum fine being well over $100,000. OSHA officials base fines on the type of violation, size of employer, and past history of infractions. Employers have the right to contest any violation, and a decision is made within a reasonable time period (as determined by OSHA officials). OSHA does not close an audit until all violations have been corrected, and there is always a deadline for completion.

OSHA offers private sector employers a free training program that is designed to prevent injuries, illnesses, and fatalities. It is based on proactive responses to workplace health and safety issues using employer and employee involvement. Employers who elect to undergo training in this program are protected from citations and fines, but they must correct all violations found by OSHA officials.
In addition to the free training program, OSHA also offers a wealth of web-based health and safety information that is free of charge to everyone. Topics discussed include compliance requirements, employee rights, and employer responsibilities. Most private sector companies use this information rather undergo the free training program.

Unfortunately, OSHA has been heavily criticized since its inception by a wide variety of individuals and organizations. Employer criticisms include unfair treatment of employees, lack of inspector qualifications, and unnecessary fines. Watchdog organizations complaints typically revolve around the fact there is not enough criminal prosecution...especially when a fatality results from negligent actions. Another watchdog complaint is that new regulations take much too long to implement. Lengthy implementation periods are not unusual for government organizations, but OSHA stands out from the rest because people's health and well-being are at stake.

OSHA is a fairly complex government agency with an extensive list of rules and regulations. This organization could be discussed and debated for hundreds of hours and thousands of pages could be written about it in a comprehensive book. However, OSHA is not the focus of this book...as is discussed in the next section.

Scope

This book focuses on safety risks in manufacturing facilities. It extracts bits and pieces from OSHA regulations and uses them to designate and explain major safety issues that manufacturing employees encounter on a regular basis. It is intended to give a better understanding of why these issues exist so manufacturers can begin the process of correcting them. This book is a good reference for people interested in safety in manufacturing plants, and it can be referred back to when needed. That being said, it is time to discuss specific safety risks in manufacturing.

These risks include:

- Machinery
- Chemicals
- Lockout/Tagout
- Confined Spaces

- Sabotage
- Training
- Extremes
- Electrical
- Substance abuse
- Material handling
- Housekeeping
- Structure

The following section discusses the above risks in more detail while providing reasons for their existence.

Risks

Manufacturing employees have always been challenged by safety risks, but these risks have decreased quite a bit over the years. One simply needs to read Upton Sinclair's 1906 book *The Jungle* for a realistic look at safety in manufacturing plants of the past. The *Constitutional Rights Foundation* notes the following in regard to Chicago meat packing plants mentioned in Sinclair's book:

> "Jurgis saw men in the pickling room with skin diseases. Men who used knives on the sped-up assembly lines frequently lost fingers. Men who hauled 100-pound hunks of meat crippled their backs. Workers with tuberculosis coughed constantly and spit blood on the floor. Right next to where the meat was processed, workers used primitive toilets with no soap and water to clean their hands. In some areas, no toilets existed, and workers had to urinate in a corner. Lunchrooms were rare, and workers ate where they worked."

Based on the above quote, it is rather easy to see that the United States has come a long way in terms of health and safety in manufacturing. However, regardless of the improvement, safety is still a concern in manufacturing...and this will likely always be the case. Many facilities hire safety managers to make sure their manufacturing operations meet or exceed OSHA standards, and this is expensive for those organizations. Time and money are required to train employees, implement policies, and arrange workplaces so they conform to existing standards. Safety is an important issue, and employers have grasped the concept that employee health and welfare is paramount.

Below are 12 major safety risks associated with manufacturing facilities along with a discussion on why those risks exist.

Machinery

Manufacturing plants need machines because they enable companies to produce far more products than they could ever make using human labor alone. For this reason, machinery in manufacturing facilities will always be a present in the environment.

Unfortunately, the downside to machinery is the constant threat of operator injury...or even death in extreme cases. Machines have chains, pulleys, sprockets, and other moving parts that pose safety threats to the operators and employees in the immediate vicinity. One example is a finger, hand, or entire limb being severed by s sharp edge. Another example is hair becoming caught in rotating parts causing scalping or entanglement. A third example is an air hose breaking off resulting in an employee losing an eye. A complete list of potential harm to employees is too extensive and graphic for this book, but the point is that machines are very capable of injuring workers. That being said, the following adds to the likelihood that machines will cause harm:

- **Disrepair** - It should not come as a surprise that machines in manufacturing facilities break down over time. They get repetitive use, for up to 24 hours a day, and their demise is ultimately inevitable. What might be surprising is the fact that these machines are often not repaired when they do break down as long...as they continue to function. They are left to deteriorate even further with operators doing their best to keep them running. This type of environment sets the stage for injuries as employees tamper with machine parts that they know little or nothing about. For this reason, disrepair of machinery is a major safety concern that often times does not receive the attention that it deserves.

- **Age** - Along the same lines of disrepair, the age of machinery also poses a safety hazard. Some machines have been properly maintained, but they are simply too old to function as designed or intended. They become worn out and can no longer be repaired...and this causes safety issues that only get worse with time. Father time is relentless, and machines that become too old pose the potential to harm employees until they are removed or replaced.

- **Temporary fixes** - Most people are well aware that temporary fixes are not the answers to problems because they are not permanent solutions. However, temporary fixes are quite common in manufacturing facilities because they allow employees to keep working. Also known as "band-aids," these repairs are sometimes more dangerous than doing nothing at all because employees believe their machines are working properly. Workers go back to their normal mode of operation, only to have the temporary fix break without warning....and they end up getting injured. Temporary fixes can cause major problems in terms of worker safety, but, unfortunately, this is not understood by some leaders of manufacturing facilities.

- **Noise** - Many people find noise to be annoying, but it has the potential to cause far more severe problems in manufacturing facilities. The most obvious issue is that it can damage employees' hearing unless they are wearing some type of ear protection. Over time, hearing damage can become permanent causing workers problems in all aspects of their jobs. However, less obvious safety threats from noise also exist. When workers lose their sense of hearing, they are unaware of the danger that lurks in manufacturing plants. They cannot hear warning signals that indicate safety issues, and this exposes them to safety problems without an opportunity to react appropriately to protect their well-being. Additionally, noise can interfere with verbal communication which increases the chance of accidents due to the inability to hear what others are saying.

- **Lack of preventative maintenance** - Preventative maintenance is critical for manufacturers who want to keep their machines operating effectively and efficiently. Regularly scheduled maintenance prevents machines from failing, and it also protects machine operators. In fact, preventative maintenance is one of the most common reasons that operators get hurt. Machines can injure or kill people in seconds...especially if they are not maintained.

  Unfortunately, some maintenance personnel in manufacturing plants cannot seem to fit preventative maintenance into their schedules. Yes, these individuals are very busy. Sometimes they have more work to do than any other department, working seven days a week...but this is not a valid excuse for not performing preventative maintenance. An example where preventative maintenance is lacking is a machine with blades used for cutting material. If these blades are not routinely sharpened, they become dull and tear rather than cut. A safety hazard is created when employees need to reach into the machine to pull apart the material because it was not cleanly cut. This type of injury can easily be avoided if the blades are properly maintained.

- **Lack of money** - Many manufacturers have good intentions when it comes to safety. They truly want to protect their employees from injury by using machinery that poses minimal risk for harming humans. However, regardless of their intent, they fall short on safety goals due to limited financial resources. They find themselves in situations where they simply do not have the money to invest in machinery upkeep.

  Unfortunately, lack of money is quite common in manufacturing plants, especially when those plants are small or new. Most people who have opened manufacturing operations are well aware that machinery can be quite costly to operate, and safety is an area where short-term savings can be realized. However, manufacturing leaders need to think about safeguarding machines before the potential for injury becomes reality and their long-term financial situations become dismal. In terms of forgoing machine safety, a penny saved is not always a penny earned.

- **Lack of technology** - It is virtually impossible for manufacturers to keep up with all of the latest machinery technology. Change is continual and managers who stay abreast of it cannot afford to implement every upgrade. However, some technology needs to be looked at more seriously than others...especially when employee safety is involved. Modern advances are sometimes geared toward protecting employees, and these advances warrant special attention from manufacturers. In terms of safety, technology can be a lifesaver.

Chemicals

Most manufacturing plants use chemicals in some capacity. The chemicals can be purchased for servicing reasons, such as those used for cleaning equipment, or they can be a necessary part of the machine or its parts, such as the acid found in batteries. Regardless of the method of entry into the facility, these chemicals present safety threats to employees working around them.

The following are major areas in manufacturing facilities where chemical risks are present:

- **Sanitation** - Most manufacturing facilities need to be cleaned, but some need more cleaning than others. For example, pharmaceutical and food plants need to be frequently cleaned. Floors, walls, ceilings, equipment, and machinery must be cleaned and sanitized in order to prevent any type of contamination.

  The majority of cleaning that takes place in manufacturing plants requires the use of chemicals. These chemicals can be strong caustic or alkaline based products that have the potential to injure employees who come in contact with them. For this reason, cleaning chemicals are a safety risk for employees.

- **Laboratories** - Anyone who is familiar with chemistry laboratories understands chemicals are needed for the different types of analyses that are performed. Testing requires different strengths of potentially harmful chemicals that are handled on a daily basis by laboratory technicians. These technicians are typically educated and trained for their jobs, but accidents can and do happen...and this is why laboratories present a safety concern for the employees working in them.

- **Maintenance** - Similar to laboratory employees, maintenance personnel frequently handle potentially hazardous chemicals. They work with various types of Freon, ammonia, paint, oil, gas, lubricants, and other chemicals to service refrigeration units, boilers, vehicles, and machinery. A well-known example is the gasoline used as fuel for engines. It has the potential to catch on fire or explode if not handled properly, and this makes it a safety threat for maintenance employees.

- **Water** (chemicals in drinking water) - Some manufacturers treat water with chlorine, softeners, or pH altering chemicals to make it more suitable for their needs. If the concentrations of these chemicals become excessive, then employees' health can be at risk. This safety threat is rather minor, but it does exist and warrants mention in this section.

The following also pose threats for manufacturers that house chemicals:

- **Improper labeling** - Chemicals that are not properly labeled pose huge safety threats for employees in manufacturing workplaces because those employees risk injury regardless of the precautions taken. They are not aware of the chemicals they are using...making it virtually impossible to prevent misuse. If misuse occurs, then the well-being of everyone is jeopardized, thereby creating a situation that can have devastating effects.

  The potential consequences for wrongly labeled chemicals are very serious, and that is why improper labeling is considered an important safety threat in manufacturing facilities.

- **Improper usage** - Proper labeling of chemicals does not prevent improper usage. All the signage, instructions, warnings, and training are useless if employees choose to use chemicals wrongly. For example, a worker might believe that mixing two chemical cleaners will produce one "super cleaner" that has twice the strength. This might be true, but it can also cause toxic fumes or explosions.

Improper usage also results from inadequate training. Employees are at serious risk if they have not been shown how, when, where, and why they should use chemicals in their facilities. Much can be written about the training and improper usage, and that is discussed in the training section of this book.

Unfortunately, improper usage of chemicals in manufacturing facilities can be intentional. Perpetrators fully understand the damage that chemicals can cause, and they used them to attack others. When this happens, it is considered an act of terrorism that threatens the safety of all employees.

- **Improper storage** - One might question why improper storage of chemicals in manufacturing plants poses safety risks to employees. After all, these chemicals are not being used or handled...so what is the problem? In reality, improperly stored chemicals present a few different types of safety hazards. For example, they can leak and contaminate the ground or surrounding water. This poses a major threat to employees' drinking water, and it also threatens everyone else who drinks from the same water source. Leaks that that do not contaminate the ground or water also pose threats if employees come in contact with the chemical. An example is a battery that leaks acid. Employees who touch that acid by mistake can experience chemical burns.

  Another issue involving chemical storage involves damage. In busy manufacturing facilities, damage to inventory is inevitable. Chemicals are part of a plant's inventory and they can be damaged by pallet jacks or forklifts. If this happens, the surrounding areas become contaminated. Fire is now a safety risk and, in extreme cases, so are explosions.

  Properly stored chemicals are typically not a safety risk for employees, but problems result when they are not stored properly. Management needs to realize the potential for problems here and act accordingly by using responsible chemical storage protocols.

Lockout/Tagout

Lockout/Tagout programs are needed by manufacturers because they assure all energy sources of equipment and/or machinery are locked out during service work or maintenance work; thereby protecting employees from being harmed by accidental activation or release of stored energy. Energy sources typically include the following:

- Electricity
- Gas
- Gravity
- Hydraulic
- Kinetic

- Pneumatic
- Thermal

Lockout/Tagout devices are unique because they are individually numbered and keyed. Many times these devices they are assigned to specific employees so no one else can open them once they are locked. They are also red in color so they can be easily identified. For safety reasons, these devices have one purpose...to lock out machines or equipment. They cannot be used for locking anything else (bikes, lockers, etc.).

The following are situations where Lockout/Tagout is required:

- **Equipment cleaning or jam-clearing tasks** - When a machine or piece of equipment is stopped for cleaning, clearing, or adjusting.
- **Equipment Repair** - When a repair is being performed...including machinery and equipment from which a guard or other safety device has been removed.
- **Installation** - When machinery or equipment is being installed.
- **Electrical Repair** - When work other than testing is to be performed on an electrical circuit.

In contrast, the following are situations where Lockout/Tagout is not required:

- **Minor tool changes** - When a stop button is used to control unexpected motion during the change or adjustment and when the start button is both visible and under the employee's immediate control.
- **Routine or repetitive minor servicing** - When activities take place during normal production and the work is performed using alternative protective measures that provide effective employee protection.
- **Cord and plug connected equipment** - When the equipment or machine is unplugged and under the exclusive control of the employee performing the service or maintenance.
- **Repair, troubleshooting, and set-up adjustments** - When work on energized equipment or machinery must be done with the machine energized.

When Lockout/Tagout is required, a procedure is necessary. An example of the procedure for a manufacturing facility is as follows:

1. Identify the types of energy sources that need to be isolated on the targeted machinery or equipment.
2. Notify all affected employees about the Lockout/Tagout taking place on the targeted machinery or equipment.
3. Verify the surrounding area is clear and make sure employees are not working on the targeted machinery or equipment.
4. Shut down the targeted machinery or equipment using emergency stops, switches, PLCs, disconnects, and corded plug-in types.
5. Verify all targeted machinery or equipment start/stop locations are powered down and all stored energy is released.
6. Apply Lockout/Tagout devices to targeted machinery or equipment.

7. Verify Lockout/Tagout devices are properly secured on the targeted machinery or equipment.
8. Perform the service or maintenance on the targeted machinery or equipment.
9. Notify affected employees of the Lockout/Tagout is being removed from the on the targeted machinery or equipment.
10. Verify the surrounding area is clear, employees are not working, and safety guards are in place on the targeted machinery or equipment.
11. Remove Lockout/Tagout devices and re-energize the targeted equipment or machinery.

Lockout/tagout programs have prevented injuries and saved lives in many instances. Based on this, it is rather manufacturing employees are at risk if Lockout/Tagout devices are not in place as required by OSHA law. Unfortunately, many manufacturers have good Lockout/Tagout programs written, but they are generally disregarded and not taken seriously by the workforce. This problem results from management inefficiency, and it will not correct itself without intervention from those in higher positions. That being said, the biggest safety issue concerning Lockout/Tagout programs is not designing or writing them; it is the failure to implement, maintain, and enforce them...and that is why they are a major safety concern in manufacturing facilities.

Confined spaces

Confined spaces are a reality in manufacturing plants that cannot be avoided. They pose a safety risk list for employees because limited air and escape routes create potentially deadly situations for workers trapped inside them. Unfortunately, some employees do not realize or acknowledge the danger involved even though their lives could be on the line in emergency situations.

Confined spaces are sometimes confused with small spaces. The size of the area does not necessarily make a space confined. In order for a space to be considered confined, it must meet the following criteria:

- It must be large enough for a person to fit into and perform work.
- It must have restricted entry and exit points.
- It must not be designed for continuous occupancy.
- It must have the potential for injury due to the enclosure.

Based on the above criteria, confined spaces in manufacturing facilities include tanks, silos, containers, chambers, bins, pits, crawl spaces, and ceiling gaps. All of these spaces are necessary for manufacturing, and they create situations where injury is possible. Atmospheric issues including fumes, gas, dust, smoke, and lack of oxygen all pose safety issues. For example, flour storage silos in bakeries pose safety risks because combustible dust is very explosive when suspended in the air. Along the same lines, employees working in septic tanks or sewers are exposed to a hazardous gas called methane that carries a risk of exploding... so it is not safe to perform tasks such as welding. Methane also displaces oxygen and makes it difficult to breathe.

Oxygen is an interesting concept in confined spaces because too much or too little can create a safety hazard. Too little oxygen is a result of it being displaced by another gas causing people to experience breathing problems. They can pass out and experience brain damage or death without emergency treatment. Excessive oxygen increases the risk of fire or explosion because some materials spontaneously burn in enriched oxygen conditions.

Flooding is also a threat in confined spaces. For example, water can enter causing people to drown. Unfortunately, water might be the best case scenario in terms of flooding. Chemical floods can cause skin burns and suffocation....two very unpleasant effects for the workers who experience them.

Maintenance and sanitation workers typically experience the most safety risks in confined spaces because they need to perform some of their job functions in these areas. For example, a maintenance worker might need to need to go down into a sewer to repair a broken drain. Along the same lines, a sanitation worker might need to be lowered into a flour silo in order to properly clean it.

The worst part about confined spaces is the fact that many times employees do not realize the danger when entering them. They do not take any precautions and unknowingly proceed as if everything is normal. In a relatively short period of time, they find themselves in an unsafe situation...with the potential to be life-threatening.

Sabotage

Sabotage is the most unfortunate safety risk associated with manufacturing because it is intentional, and it has the potential to become a huge nightmare for everyone involved. It damages physical assets, people, and reputations of organizations. The resulting domino effect of negative public perception is hard to overcome, and it can cause some manufacturers to go out of business.

Sabotage will exist as long as employees are unhappy with their employers...which means it will likely never disappear. An example of sabotage is a disgruntled employee who plants a bomb after being fired from a manufacturing facility. Property is destroyed and employees are injured...all due to the unhappiness of one individual. However, the problem not does stop with the explosion because the after effects can also be destructive. When this story reaches the news, it can cause the public to view the company in a negative light due to their action of firing the employee or their lack of action from preventing the sabotage. Regardless of the reason for the negative perception, the manufacturer's reputation is damaged. This puts them in a difficult situation because time and effort are needed to gain back the trust and respect of their customers and the general public.

In terms of safety, sabotage threatens employees' physical and mental well-being. Physically they can be injured and, in extreme cases, those injuries can be fatal. In fact, some sabotage is conducted with the deliberate intent of killing people. However, employees who experience sabotage are subject to more than just physical pain. Their mental health can also be negatively impacted because they have to deal with the thought of what happened. Emotional scars are not always quick to heal...and sometimes they never completely disappear.

Training

Production employees need training in order to understand how to do their jobs properly. Part of that training involves safety because, without safety, employees risk injury. They enter unknown territory and are unsure how to prevent potentially dangerous situations...and how to get out of those situations if they become a reality.

Training starts with showing workers how to properly operate equipment. This involves understanding body positioning, ergonomics, fatigue, distractions, safety features, and shutoffs in the event of an emergency. This might seem rather basic or simple to some readers of this book, but many times it is the exact opposite. In crisis situations, employees have only seconds to react, and often times they do not react properly in terms of limiting injury to themselves or others.

Manufacturer's need to realize that proper safety training cannot be conducted if the trainers do not possess the required skills to teach others. Obviously, those skills involve understanding plant operations and the machinery being used. Trainers need to be able to teach employees how to behave to prevent unsafe situations and how to act in the event of an emergency. However, one often overlooked skill of instructors is their ability to assess the people being trained. The need to understand the skills and capabilities of the plant employees and alter the course design based on a well-thought analysis. For example, skilled tradesman have typically already had safety training, so they will have a good comprehension of the material being presented. Conversely, that level of comprehension is not always the same for new employees or those who have never had any formal training. These individuals might need extra time and explanation to absorb the information...and the trainer needs to realize and react to this need.

Common barriers to proper training of manufacturing employees include the following;

- **Language** - This is one of the biggest barriers so it deserves to be mentioned first. Many production facilities employ immigrants whose first language is not English. This results in misunderstanding and lack of comprehension when safety training is conducted only in English. By no means does this mean these employees are "dumb" or incapable of learning. They may be very smart and eager to learn...but that learning is only accomplished in their native tongues.

  Potential solution - Manufacturers can hire translators if the money is available to do so. However, if money is a concern, then coworkers who speak the same language can be utilized to translate. Additionally, written documents can be translated for free on various internet websites. These translations are typically not perfect, but the information that they do provide is better than nothing at all.

- **Lack of information** - Regardless of the comprehension or understanding of the trainees, they will not learn what they need to know if information is left out. Some trainers assume the trainees already have an understanding of a particular concept, so they skip over it and move into the next part of the course. This might not be common, but it does occur and that is why it is listed as a barrier to training. There is an old saying that states "never assume anything." This saying has great application in safety training because improper assumptions can lead to injury or death.

Potential solution - Assume employees know very little in terms of safety. Trainers should start with the easiest aspects of training and work up to more complex topics. Although this might be boring for some of the participants, it could prevent injury and/or save lives.

- **Lack of clarity** - Many employees are afraid of looking "dumb" or "stupid" in front of their coworkers, so they avoid asking questions for a better understanding of what they are attempting to learn. This presents a situation that does not resolve itself...and trainees leave without having a full understanding of what they have been taught.

Potential solution - Smaller training groups often help employees feel more comfortable asking questions that they believe might embarrass them in front of their co-workers. Another solution is to allow employees an opportunity to post anonymous questions during the training that are only seen by the trainer. Privacy is a concern of some trainees, and that concern needs to be taken into consideration in order to assure proper learning.

- **Lack of visual** - Whoever coined the term "a picture is worth a thousand words" was one hundred percent correct. However, some trainers fail to realize this little gem of advice. Instead, they work their way through presentations using lecture only, choosing to describe the subject matter rather than showing an image. Visual aids, in some shape or form, are often underused by trainers....and this hampers the ability of the trainees to learn the material.

Potential solution - Visual aids must be used during safety presentations. Videos are great, but they are not the only option. Signs can be posted in the classroom, handouts can be issued, posters can be hung, and pictures can be distributed. The advantages of visual aids cannot be underestimated because they work wonders for helping trainees comprehend and understand.

- **Lack of follow-up** - This barrier is unique because it takes place after the training is completed. Once safety procedures have been put in place, they need to be followed up on to make sure they are successful. Management often overlooks follow-up by failing to post reminders in the plant or neglecting to see if the training is working.

Potential solution - Signs can be posted around machinery to point out specific safety procedures, posters can be hung on walls throughout the plant to promote general safety, and periodic emails or memos can be sent to employees to remind them about the importance of safety. Additionally, supervisors need to walk around and make mental notes of what is happening in terms of safety. Are employees following established protocols? If not, then they might need to be retrained verbally or in a more formal setting.

Extremes

The first type of extreme that warrants discussion as a safety risk is temperature. Hot and cold temperatures pose major safety threats to employees if those employees are not cautious.

Extreme temperatures can come from the air, a surface, a product, or machinery. Regardless of the source, temperatures can be extremely hot or cold and present safety risks for employees. Extreme cold can cause hypothermia or frostbite. Workers can lose feeling in their feet hands....and that feeling might never come back. Extreme heat can result in employees fainting or experiencing strokes...and their condition can be made worse because they are wearing personal protective equipment that keeps the heat in their bodies.

The following are examples of the four different types of hot and cold extremes noted in the previous paragraph:

> **Air** - Air temperature in a manufacturing facility can vary greatly depending on the type of operation. For example, a foundry-based manufacturing plant is often very hot while a frozen food manufacturer has some very cold areas. In both cases, the temperature of the air is a threat to the safety of employees exposed to it. Workers wear personal protective equipment such as face shields, insulated clothing, and gloves to protect themselves...but the threat of exposure is always present.

> **Surface** – Surfaces can reach extreme temperatures based on their function. For example, the dies used for forming steel in a bolt manufacturing plant get very hot after the melted metal is deposited in them. Employees who touch these dies risk severe burns, so they need to avoid contact.

> **Product** – Products made in manufacturing facilities also reach extreme temperatures. For example, hard candy produced in a confectionary reaches very high temperatures. Since this product must be handled while hot in order to "pull" it into specific shapes, it presents a safety risk and proper gloves must be used.

> **Machinery** – Motors in machines get very hot...to the extent that air, water, or some other substance is required to cool them. For example, the motor on a packaging machine in a pharmaceutical manufacturer reaches dangerously high temperatures that pose a safety threat to employees working near it.

> Machinery also uses steam. Steam is so hot that it can literally peel the skin off of a person. Employees who do not take precautionary measures can end up badly injured.

The second type of extreme refers to pneumatics...more commonly known as air pressure. Air pressure is needed in manufacturing facilities for equipment and machinery, and this will likely never change. However, compressed air is dangerous because it is strong enough to cause many different types of injuries. It is much stronger than many people might think, and it is capable of blinding someone if direct contact is made with their eyes. It can also pierce or tear skin, and the "squealing" noise has the potential to cause hearing damage.

Compressed air is something that should never be taken lightly in terms of safety. It is needed in manufacturing facilities, but dangers associated with it are often taken much too lightly by employees exposed to it. Air pressure is an extreme safety risk, and it needs to be dealt with as such.

The last extreme risk discussed in this book involves ventilation. The concern here is a lack of ventilation and the resulting fumes that cause safety threats. Sometimes no amount of ventilation will prevent the fumes...such as those encountered in an ammonia leak. However, fumes from an ammonia leak are easily detected by employees, causing them to exit quickly. Much more dangerous are fumes that cannot be detected, such as carbon monoxide. Carbon monoxide has killed thousands of workers in different industries, and it is no stranger to manufacturing. It is a colorless and odorless gas that overtakes employees with no warning. If this happens, the results can be deadly..and that is why ventilation is listed as an extreme safety hazard.

Electrical

Anyone who has witnessed an electrical fire understands the safety concerns involved with this power source. Fire can result from faulty wiring or a variety of electrical code violations...including unauthorized items stored in electrical rooms. Regardless of the reason, fire starting from electrical issues can spread to other areas, and it has the potential to injure or kill people.

Since electricity is the blood of most manufacturing plants, it presents a major safety risk for the employees who work around it. Shortcuts are often the biggest concern due to the constant pressure to keep production running. "Temporary" fixes become permanent over time, and they are never thought about again until they break or something drastic occurs. For example, extension cords are sometimes used to convey power rather than following the proper code and hard wiring the system. This works great until those cords are damaged....and then they become a safety hazard.

It must be noted that many safety concerns involving electricity can be prevented by using proper lockout/tagout procedures. If there is no power or stored energy, then people will not be injured by electrical currents, shorts, or surges during service or maintenance. However, lockout/tagout is not used during normal production...and this is when the majority of potential safety issues involving electricity become reality. For example, if production employees do not know that a wire is live, they might not use precautions and end up getting shocked. A 110-volt shock can produce little more than discomfort, but a 220 volt or 440-volt shock can be deadly.

Managers of manufacturing facilities need to take the time to follow electrical code or risk injuring their workforces. This means production cannot always be put first; it might need to take a backseat to safety. This might be financially painful, but it could save the lives of employees.

Substance abuse

Drug and alcohol abuse occurs all over the world, and there is little indication of this stopping. Some manufacturing employees prefer to get drunk or high before performing their jobs...especially if their jobs are repetitive or mundane such as many of those found in production facilities. Other people become addicted to drugs, and they find themselves in need of that drug in order to avoid withdrawal. Regardless of the reason, substance abusers cannot perform their jobs at peak levels due to drugs or alcohol in their systems.

Interestingly, many peoples' drug and alcohol addictions do not start illegally. They take a prescribed painkiller or psychotic drug for a legitimate medical ailment and end up with an addiction. In short, they start by seeking the help of a licensed doctor and eventually turn to the unlawful activity of the streets in search of the same drug to feed their addiction needs.

Employees who are under the influence of drugs or alcohol are a safety threat to everyone in the workplace. This is especially true for manufacturing workers who deal with equipment or machinery because a dangerous situation can result due to operator impairment. Safety issues involving equipment or machinery can result with little or no warning, leaving the affected employees virtually defenseless to the harm that they are about to encounter.

The worse part about injuries that result from substance abuse is the fact that many of them could have been prevented. Employees should be monitored for drug usage via random testing...and taken off their jobs for treatment when results indicate the potential for injury to themselves or others. This is a proactive, rather than reactive, response to a safety concern that could prevent a lot of pain and suffering for employees along with unnecessary expenses for manufacturers.

Material handling

Material handling has been a safety risk for manufacturers since the very beginning. Material always needs to be moved from one area to another resulting in ample opportunity for injury. Unfortunately, it is often the innocent bystander that is injured during material handling incidents. They get in the way of the employee moving the material and end up getting hurt.

The biggest safety risk in material handling is the use of powered transportation. Power jacks have the potential to run over employees or trap them against walls, knock over shelving or bays of product, and cause damage to machines that make them unsafe to operate. Forklifts pose even more threats because power and speed are increased. Add the elevated forks that have the potential to "stick" people, and it is not hard to envision the safety hazards that they create.

Much of the risk involved with material handling can be eliminated with simple safety procedures. Employees moving material need to slow down and pay attention to where they are going and what is in their path. They also need to exercise caution in terms of speed because it is much easier to react to a dangerous situation when moving slowly. Ultimately, safety with material handling boils down to common sense...something that workers should use without being told to do so.

Housekeeping

Housekeeping is a rather broad term that refers to making sure the manufacturing "house" is in proper order. It involves making sure that plants are properly maintained, cleaned, and kept free of debris and clutter so employees are not exposed to unsafe situations. For example, slippery floors create a risk of workers falling and getting injured. If these floors are slippery because they are wet, then signs should be posted to warn people of the danger. If the floors are naturally slippery, then some type of grit should be put down. Regardless of the reason for the problem, it needs to be controlled...and good housekeeping is the solution.

Another example of the need for good housekeeping includes clutter. Manufacturers tend to hold on to obsolete or unused machines, parts, and equipment because they might be needed in the future. When maintenance personnel run out of storage space, they infringe upon other areas that were not designed for storage...and this is where the problems begin. Clutter creates safety hazards because employees have to navigate around it to do their jobs. It also impairs workers views of where they are going, and they can hit someone or something due to their lack of vision. In short, employees who are not careful can injure themselves or others. For this reason, clutter needs to be avoided.

A third example of the need for good housekeeping involves plant maintenance. This should not be confused with machine maintenance because it refers to the upkeep of the physical plant, not the upkeep of machinery and equipment. Damaged cement, broken doors, and crumbling wall or ceilings all present safety hazards for employees working in the facility. Without proper upkeep, employees can trip and fall or get hit by falling debris. Plant managers need to understand this risk and react accordingly by keeping their plants in good condition.

The last example of housekeeping is cleaning of the facility. Improper cleaning results in debris being left in the plant. This is similar to clutter, but it does not involve machines, parts, and equipment. Instead, it involves scraps, waste, garbage, and other matter that should be picked up and thrown in the trash. Employees exposed to these types of conditions can injure themselves or others simply because they are trying to avoid the debris by moving around it or stepping over it. The simple fix to this housekeeping problem is to hire a janitorial staff that keeps the plant clean...something that many plants avoid due to the expense. However, the cost of injuries can far exceed the cost of a janitorial staff in a relatively short period of time.

Structure

This refers to the structure that leadership needs to implement and maintain in a manufacturing facility. Managers and supervisors must understand their roles in terms of safety. They need to involve employees in the process so those employees are aware of safety issues, and they also need to enforce the safety rules and regulations that are in place.

Employees are considered to be involved when they are aware of their surroundings and the safety risks involved with those surroundings. These risks include:

- Understanding the safeties on the machines they operate

- Understanding the power sources on the machines they operate
- Understanding how to perform lockout/tagout on the machines they operate
- Understanding the personal protective equipment needed for the machines they operate

Employees are also considered involved when they understand the work rules put in place by their employers and the consequences for not adhering to these rules. The following are examples of safety rules that manufacturing facilities might have in place:

- *All injuries must be reported to management as soon as possible.*

  The key word in this rule is "all." Some injuries are overlooked when they are considered minor, but this should never happen. Employees must report every injury, regardless of its severity, so it can be documented and properly addressed. Anything less can result in problems that lead to health and/or financial consequences.

- *Drugs or alcohol are not allowed on the premises unless prescribed and authorized for use on the job by a licensed medical doctor.*

  As might be expected, alcohol and illegal drugs are strictly forbidden. However, an important part of this rule involves the restrictions written by prescribing doctors of legal drugs. These restrictions must clearly state that the affected employees can operate their machinery while on the medication...or else those employees are not allowed to work.

- *Safeties and guards must always be in place, in good working condition, and never overridden.*

  Machine guards and safeties are put in place for a reason...to protect operators and employees in the immediate area. For example, they prevent people from being cut by blades, exposed to extreme temperatures, or caught in moving parts. Safeties and guards should only be removed for maintenance or service after the affected machines have been locked out. If safeties or guards are damaged, then that damage needs to be immediately reported to management where it can be appropriately addressed. This prevents employees from being injured.

- *Personal protective equipment must be worn by all employees when applicable.*

  Regardless of the safeties and guards in place, many different types of machinery and equipment in manufacturing plants require employees to wear personal protective equipment to prevent injury. This equipment includes specially designed goggles, glasses, gloves, shoes, boots, aprons, arm guards, and face shields. Many employees work for long periods of time without the need for protection from this equipment...but it is there in case something happens that jeopardizes their physical well-being.

- *Horseplay and roughhousing are not allowed.*

  Employers want their employees to enjoy their jobs. After all, workers who enjoy their jobs are much more likely to remain employed at their current organization, and they will look forward to work rather than dreading it. In fact, "having fun at work" has recently become a topic of interest in organizational discussions. However, that fun is not acceptable when horseplay occurs in manufacturing facilities. Essentially, horseplay is some type of physical activity performed by employees in order to get a break from their routine daily activities. This might be acceptable for some organizations, but it has no place in manufacturing plants. Employees who fail to focus on their jobs risk injuring themselves or their co-workers. This statement is not based on some type of academic theory...it is a fact because workers have been injured in manufacturing facilities while engaging in horseplay in many different instances.

- *Forklifts can only be driven by employees possessing proper permits.*

  As noted earlier, forklifts are quite capable of injuring people if proper care is not exercised by the drivers. For this reason, employees must pass a physical and written test to receive a permit to operate forklifts. Without this permit, employees are not allowed to drive these types of transportation vehicles...with no exceptions.

Summary

This book is a reference for 12 important safety risks in manufacturing. It describes these risks and explains why they exist. These risks include the following:

- Machinery
- Chemicals
- Lockout/Tagout
- Confined spaces
- Sabotage
- Training
- Extremes
- Electrical
- Substance abuse
- Material handling
- Housekeeping
- Structure

The above risks are continuing to grow in importance as manufacturing leaders all over the world realize the value of their employees and the significance of protecting those employees' health and safety.

Congratulations! You now understand more about important safety risks associated with manufacturing....and this book can be used as a reference to look back on those risks whenever it is needed.